Praise for *The Addicted Brain*

"Once again, Dr. Cass has written an easy-to-read, easy-to-understand book about a not-so-easy subject. She performs a huge public health service by tackling one of today's major crises, and brings hope to the patients and their families. Doctors should consider this recommended reading if they put themselves out as addiction experts."

—Garry M Vickar, MD, FRCPC, Distinguished Life Fellow, American Psychiatric Association; Lecturer, Washington University Dept. of Psychiatry, St. Louis; Professor and Clinical Chair, Dept. of Psychiatry, St Matthews University

As owner of one of the leading treatment centers of the country, I've been blessed with the opportunity to see hundreds of suffering addicts recover. Dr. Cass is an expert in the addiction treatment field. We use many of the principles contained in this book to treat our patients. Anyone whose life is touched by addiction MUST read this book! Dr. Cass delivers a comprehensive picture of the disease of addiction, and what those suffering need to do to get well.

—Jim Marshall, co-founder of Serenity Springs Recovery Center, New Smyrna Beach, FL

As founder of the premier holistic addiction treatment center in the country, I can unequivocably state that Dr. Cass knows both her science and clinical information. This book explains the underlying biochemistry of addiction: how addiction is not simply a matter of willpower, but of influencing your brain chemicals with specific nutrients to restore balance, stop cravings, and make you feel normal again.

—John Giordano, Doctor of Human Letters, CCJS, MAC, CAP, founder of The National Institute for Holistic Addiction Studies (NIFHAS)—www.holisticaddictioninfo.com

The Addicted Brain

And How to Break Free

Using Natural

Supplements

HYLA CASS, MD

Better Balance Books
Marina del Rey, CA

For wholesale orders, contact **office@cassmd.com**
and put ADDICTION BOOK on subject line.

Contents

Introduction

This book is about addiction: yours, that of your friends and relatives, and really, of our society as a whole.

For starters, my approach to addiction is *not* that of mainstream or conventional medical care. No surprise here! I have been alarmed at the growing problems of addiction in all areas (food, drugs, medications, and activities) leading to a great deal of suffering by those directly and indirectly affected. The way it's being treated, or not treated, is equally upsetting, which led me to write and speak on natural approaches to addiction whenever I can.

I'm excited to share this information with you, so you can understand how addiction works insidiously on your brain, body, and every aspect of your life, and how you can take back control – or help someone else who has lost their way here.

I have spent many years in medical practice, helping to repair the damage done by poor food choices, unhealthy substances, and inadequate medical care to treat it. Here's what I would like to see, and I urge you to jump on board with me to make the changes, in yourself first, in those around you, and in the broken system that knowingly or not, fosters addiction.

What is addiction and why does there seem to be an epidemic of it?

Some of the issues that seem obvious to me are:

- Rampant food addiction, fostered by the food industry, with addictiveness built into our chips and sodas and jumbo burgers, just like tobacco industry scandals. So dieting to lose weight won't help, since you'll be back eating it all (and regaining the weight) before you know it – unless you know how to change your brain!

- The scandal of prescription medicine addiction created by doctors and fostered by the pharmaceutical industry

- Mistreatment of addiction by the medical profession in 'revolving door' addiction treatment centers. I am truly tired of seeing the failure of most addiction treatment programs, with 60–90% relapse rates. The staff is often very dedicated, and the clients committed, but the process of recovery still remains very difficult.

What I'm introducing here is a deeper look 'under the hood" – i.e., a look into your brain chemistry – to see how we can correct the underlying imbalance, ending addiction rather than simply trying to control it. I'd like to see widespread availability healthy non-addictive food, far less use of medications for every little symptom, and the adoption by the addiction treatment community of the information I am presenting here.

I don't see addiction as being a sign of weakness or poor character. Rather, it's a biochemical imbalance that once corrected, can create a major shift in your brain and belief systems – and even, remove your cravings for whatever had been sought after so passionately and relentlessly. Possible? Yup.

I'll explain the underpinnings of addiction – how it starts, what occurs in your body and brain, and how to overcome it. The concepts are simple and readily applicable – in the comfort of your own home.

Ready?

SECTION 1

What You Need to Know About Addiction

Chapter 1

Understanding Addiction

You have some idea of what addiction is, either first hand (unless you can easily resist a warm Krispy Crème or double chocolate fudge cake), or having a friend or relative who suffers from it, or simply old watching movies, like *Days of Wine and Roses, Drugstore Cowboy, I'm Dancing a Fast as I Can,* or *Leaving Las Vegas.* Addiction can involve a whole range of habits, including food, tobacco, alcohol, drugs of abuse, or prescription medication, and even behaviors like gambling, pornography, or sexual activity.

Let's begin with defining addiction, including its related states, tolerance and withdrawal. If you want to dig deeper, you'll find links (click here to Wikipedia http://en.wikipedia.org/wiki/Addiction) from which I borrowed these great definitions.

Addiction, by definition, is "the continued use of a mood altering substance or behavior despite adverse consequences."

Addictions can include, but are not limited to, alcohol abuse, drug abuse, exercise abuse, sex, and gambling. Classic hallmarks of addiction include: impaired control over substances/behavior, preoccupation with substance/behavior, continued use despite consequences, and denial.

Habits and patterns associated with addiction are aimed at immediate gratification (short-term reward), coupled with delayed long-term consequences. So, to sum it up, *what seems like fun at the time has a price to pay down the road*. Old story, eh?

Sounds pretty bad, and often it is. Then we have the "lesser" addictions: the ones where we say, "I'm not addicted: I can quit whenever I want to." After reading this book, you may see more clearly that we are not as aware of our addictions as we might think.

The truth is, most addiction has profound effects both on the person involved and on those around them. It may start small, but lead to a compulsion too strong to resist. It can consume your life, with preoccupation, obsession, secrecy, denial, deception, and often destruction of lives and relationships.

"Addiction is a Brain Disease"

(a lot of big words here, but important to know)

Former Director of The National Institute on Drug Abuse (NIDA), Dr. Alan Leshner, notes in *The Journal of the American Medical Association* (JAMA-Oct. 13, 1999)

"...Advances in science have greatly increased, and in fact revolutionized, our fundamental understanding of the nature of drug abuse and addiction, and, most importantly, what to do about it.

"Although the onset of addiction begins with the voluntary act of taking drugs, the continued repetition of 'voluntary' drug taking begins to change into 'involuntary' drug taking, ultimately to the point where the behavior is driven by compulsive craving for the drug. This

13

compulsion results from a combination of factors, including in large part dramatic changes in brain function produced by prolonged drug use. This is why addiction is considered a brain disease – one with imbedded behavioral and social context aspects. Once addicted, it is almost impossible for most people to stop the spiraling cycle of addiction on their own without treatment."

I do agree, though what Dr. Leshner left unsaid is that most treatment modalities fail. We have better, natural ways to deal with addiction, as you will see.

Chapter 2
Common Myths of Addiction

After treating hundreds of substance abusers addicted to substances from alcohol, cocaine, heroin and prescription drugs, to "socially accepted drugs" like caffeine, tobacco and sugar, I have seen how a series of popular myths has often clouded the issue of addiction.

Myth 1: Compulsive use of an addictive substance is a sign of weakness or poor moral character.

Fact: You are not a weak or "bad" person. Rather, you have a brain chemistry imbalance, and moral character may have little to do with it. To prove the point, researchers took a group of rats, made them "alcoholic" then treated them with amino acids. When tested further, they had lost their cravings and addiction. Of course, human beings are more complex, have social cues, and emotional baggage – all best dealt with by a well-nourished brain.

Myth 2: Chronic addiction is a disease that can be treated with prescription drugs.

Fact: While you may have a chemical imbalance, it's not likely a Prozac or Xanax deficiency. As a psychiatrist who can prescribe drugs but chooses not to, for the most part, I deplore the standard treatment of overly medicating those in recovery, often with multiple drug "cocktails." This approach not only taxes an already overloaded system, but does not get to the root cause. It also interferes with mental and emotional rehabilitation: you can't do much in therapy or a life enhancement program when you're in a medication-induced fog. There are times in the acute withdrawal phase when a drug may be needed, but once this is over, the natural alternatives are far preferable.

Myth 3: Drugs and alcohol are the cause of substance abuse.

Fact: While using substances will increase the problem, you'll find that the underlying cause is a brain chemistry imbalance and lack of coping skills. Beneath that may be traumatic memories, resentments, shame, and guilt that need to be processed.

Myth 4: Avoiding relapse is a constant struggle for recovering substance abusers.

Fact: Once you're in balance, any craving to use is simply a sign that you need to correct your nutrition and get into positive action.

Myth 5: Relapse is part of recovery.

Fact: Relapse is just a sign of not fully embracing the solution, or not having the correct biochemical solution, even when confronted with challenges. This is when you need to be extra vigilant and follow your nutrition and lifestyle program.

Myth 6: Substance abuse runs in my family so I can't help it.

Fact: If you have a family history of substance abuse, you simply have to be more careful than most to take the appropriate nutrients. You are not a slave to your genes!

Myth 7: Addiction is due to an addictive personality.

Fact: Once the correct treatment is given, the "addictive personality" often disappears and one has the opportunity to grow (up). Social and emotional support groups, psychotherapy, and life enhancement programs are still vital, but this adds the missing piece to treatment and relapse prevention. It also allows you to begin to examine old traumas, which can themselves cause chronic (and often unconscious) stress, which continues to deplete your brain chemistry, and affect behavior.

Chapter 3
Who is an Addict?

Addiction is related to the brain chemistry, which in turn is affected by nutritional, behavioral and emotional factors. Let's begin by finding out whether you, in fact, have a real addiction problem or not. There are a series of standard questions to help figure this out, for yourself or for someone you know whom you suspect is addicted.

The standard questions are based on those from Alcoholics Anonymous and Narcotics Anonymous. Basically, the questions are asking if your life and the lives of those around you are affected in a profound way with your using or behavior, whether it's drugs, smoking, alcohol, shopping, sex, pornography, chocolate, gambling, video games, or obsession over another person. Addiction is an unhealthy obsession, accompanied by an intense "gotta-have-it" urge.

Sound familiar? Going out at a midnight because you ran out of cigarettes or are out of Jack Daniels, or just munched your last Oreo?

Behaviors such as gambling, over-exercise, and eating are included because they stimulate your brain to produce more of the pleasurable brain chemical, dopamine, giving you a "feel good" hit – often followed by feelings of guilt, shame, hopelessness, despair, failure, rejection, anxiety or humiliation.

Chapter 4
Addiction Checklist

The following is a list of standard questions to help you reflect about your habits, or of someone you are concerned about:

❏ Do you ever use or drink alone or hide your food addiction from others?

❏ Have you ever substituted one drug or addiction for another, thinking that one particular drug was the problem?

❏ Have you ever manipulated or lied to a doctor to obtain prescription drugs?

❏ Have you ever stolen drugs/alcohol or stolen to obtain drugs or alcohol?

❏ Do you regularly use a drug or drink alcohol when you wake up or when you go to bed?

❏ Have you ever taken one drug to overcome the effects of another?

❏ Do you avoid people or places that do not approve of your using drugs or drinking?

❏ Have you ever used a drug without knowing what it was or what it would do to you?

❏ Has your job or school performance ever suffered from the effects of your drug or alcohol use?

- ❑ Have you ever been arrested as a result of using drugs/alcohol?

- ❑ Have you ever lied about what or how much you use?

- ❑ Do you put the purchase of drugs or alcohol (or other addiction, such as shopping, food, games, porn) ahead of your financial responsibilities?

- ❑ Have you ever tried to stop or control your using?

- ❑ Have you ever been in a jail, hospital, or drug rehabilitation center because of your using?

- ❑ Does using interfere with your sleeping or eating?

- ❑ Does the thought of losing access to your addictive substance terrify you?

- ❑ Do you feel it is impossible for you to live without your addiction?

- ❑ Do you ever question your own sanity?

- ❑ Is your addiction use making life at home unhappy?

- ❑ Have you ever thought you couldn't fit in or have a good time without drugs or alcohol?

- ❑ Have you ever felt defensive, guilty, or ashamed about your using?

- ❑ Do you think a lot about drugs/alcohol/porn/sex/ food (whatever you are having trouble with)?

- ❑ Has using affected your sexual relationships?

- ❑ Have you ever used because of emotional pain or stress?

❑ Have you ever overdosed?

❑ Do you continue to use despite negative consequences?

Examining those questions to which you answered "yes" to will give you a good idea of whether you're addicted. And as few as one or two "yes" answers are good indicators that you may be!

Chapter 5

The Biochemical Roots

The biochemical roots of addiction lie in the same part of the brain that governs passion, love, and mental energy. Addiction has to do with an imbalance of neurotransmitters – the chemical messengers in the brain that are the molecules of thought and emotion.

The ones that we're most familiar with are dopamine, norepinephrine, serotonin, endorphins and adrenalin. Imbalances in any of these can lead to low energy, depression, and burnout, which then can drive you to look for ways of waking yourself up with whatever is on hand. Or they can lead to irritability, hyperactivity, and hypersensitivity that pulls you toward the easiest "downer" that is available. Often, it's all of these.

Your Brain: Getting the Message Across

The keys to your brain function are the chemical messengers of mind and mood called neurotransmitters. As they whizz around your brain and nervous system, they help determine how you feel.

Trillions of nerve cells, called neurons, are scattered throughout the body, but are most highly concentrated in the brain. Connecting to one another via branches called dendrites, they link together like interconnecting highways. Neurotransmitters deliver messages from one neuron to the next.

The "sending" neuron produces the neurotransmitter, propelling it toward the "receiving" neuron, across a small gap called a synapse. There it attaches to its specific receptor site, just like a key fitting into a lock. When it fits, the message is delivered – that is, the receptor is activated. An electrical signal then travels along the dendrites until it reaches the next synapse or road junction, where it triggers the release of more neurotransmitters.

Once a neurotransmitter has delivered its message, it is released from the receptor site and returns to the synapse. It might then be taken up once again into the neuron that sent it, where it can be used again, or it might be broken down and destroyed. Now that's recycling!

Each neuron, on average, makes more than 1,000 synaptic connections with other neurons. In total, there may be between 100 trillion and quadrillion synapses in the brain. Moreover, these synapses are not random but form patterns that give rise to what are called circuits in the brain. These form the basis of behavior and of mental life. How you think and feel – your mood, alertness, level of relaxation, and the state of your memory – is affected by the fine-tuned activity of these circuits, which are controlled by the interplay of the various neurotransmitters. Pretty complicated here.

One of the most awe-inspiring mysteries of brain science is how activity of neurons within circuits gives rise to behavior and, even, consciousness. There is a delicately balanced system in place involving our genetic makeup, environmental influences, memories, and neuronal health. We can, however, influence brain cell activity by supplying the right nutrients including the raw materials to produce these neurotransmitters.

To put it simply: enough of the "happy" neurotransmitters make you feel high, while deficiency will leave you feeling unmotivated or tired. They also work together like a finely tuned orchestra, and need to be in balance for you to feel just right.

While there are hundreds of neurotransmitters, the following are the main players (that we know of, at least) and their actions:

Dopamine energizes the brain, makes you motivated, focused, and on track. Not enough dopamine? You feel lethargic, apathetic and depressed, unable to focus or get moving. Caffeine, cocaine, certain addictive behaviors, and dangerous activities like reckless driving can raise dopamine levels in the brain, so if your levels are low, you may just be drawn to these activities. How do we get low in dopamine? Some of the factors here are:

- Your genes: some people are just born that way, with less dopamine or fewer receptors for it

- Poor nutrition

- Stress

- Lack of emotional connection to others.

Too much dopamine, and you're manic, losing normal inhibition and good judgment. You may turn to alcohol to chill you out. Or a doctor might prescribe tranquilizers, which have their own dangers. We have better ways.

Serotonin is another major neurotransmitter in the brain, though surprisingly, 95% of it is made in the gut, a fact than may help to explain the term "gut feeling." Serotonin regulates mood, appetite, sleep, muscle contraction and mental functions such as memory and learning. Low serotonin and you don't feel so well: depressed, anxious, tense, unable to sleep, more sensitive to pain, and craving carbs.

Stress is one factor that causes serotonin to go south, low estrogen in women is another. Most of the newer mood enhancing drugs such as *Prozac, Zoloft, Paxil, Lexapro* and *Celexa* are SSRIs – serotonin reuptake inhibitors, i.e., they prevent the drug from being taken back up, so it makes more 'hits' on the receiving cell, making it believe there is more serotonin available than there really is – till those molecules are used up and the drug stops working. Familiar? Ever experience SSRI poop-out, where the doc has to raise the dose, or add another drug? That's why.

Adrenalin is the fight-or-flight neurotransmitter, produced by the adrenal glands, which are working overtime in our modern day 24/7 lifestyles. This overdrive, along with cortisol imbalances leads to adrenal fatigue – with low energy, especially in the mid to late afternoon, or mornings when simply can't wake up, even though you think you've had sufficient sleep time. That's where the Starbucks comes in (not a great idea, though). When the stress response is on overdrive, you feel irritable, jumpy, and easily upset, with rapid heart rate, sweaty palms, and tight muscles. You may even feel nauseous.

Endorphins are the "feel good" hormones. Activities like running or even, stress, can release an abundance of endorphins, boosting the feelings of pleasure and satisfaction, so we can actually become addicted to both. Running is healthier. With a lack of endorphins, we feel apathetic, unmotivated, and tired. Life feels not worth living and you may be drawn to either stimulants or opiates. I don't recommend them.

GABA is the "chill factor" that helps us calm down. Without adequate levels of it, we are nervous, hyperactive, and most often, have trouble sleeping. We may turn to alcohol to chill us out though this can end up backfiring, with all the usual bad consequences.

When levels of these neurotransmitters are low, we feel bad: anxious, depressed, tired, and just generally uncomfortable. Wanting to feel better, we reach for what's handy, and what works: sugar, caffeine, alcohol, cocaine – whatever. Or we shop till we drop, all in an attempt to restore mental, physical or emotional energy. We'll even gamble away our family's means of support, for the momentary thrill of the pursuit of a win – a fool's journey, for sure.

The good news is that there are foods, lifestyle habits, and natural supplements can help bring these various neurotransmitters back into balance, knocking out cravings for the bad stuff. The addiction relapse rate then drops down to more like 10%.

SECTION 2

*The Many Forms
of Addiction*

Chapter 6

Overcoming Addiction

We have seen how the origins of addiction arise from the complex workings of the brain. The substances that give us pleasure – such as alcohol, coffee, sugar, cocaine, tobacco – all cause stimulation through the release of feel-good neurotransmitters.

Over time these substances can lose their "kick", requiring higher doses to maintain the feel-good effect. This occurs when the receptors for the neurotransmitters close down (called 'down-regulation') in response to the heavy bombardment of a given substance. And to complicate matters further, when you decide to stop using your substance, then you have fewer spots to receive the chemical message. Down-regulation wins every time.

The trick to overcoming addiction is to restore and regulate normal neurotransmitter balance, and maybe, even have it for the first time. Many turn to addiction in the first place in an attempt to self-treat a long-time imbalance in mood.

In this chapter, we will look at a number of addictions, including the most common legal ones – sugar, caffeine, alcohol, stimulants, relaxants, and prescription medication – and how to break free. And it doesn't have to be a frank addiction. It can be pretty subtle, so here are some of the signs:

- Do you have anxiety or depression for no apparent reason, and often related to food, especially carbs?

- Do you eat carbs, especially sugar, to feel better?

- Do you use caffeine to keep you going all day?

- How important is your after-work drink?

- Are you a smoker and don't want to or are unable to quit?

- Have you been told you have a problem with alcohol or drugs?

- Are you already aware that you have a drug, alcohol or substance abuse problem and are seeking help?

If you said "yes" to any of the questions above, you are not alone. You may not even think any of this is a problem (well, not a serious one, anyway). Read on to find out why it is, and how there is a more fulfilling way to go through life.

I believe it is possible to go through life firing on all cylinders, feeling inspired, enthusiastic, happy, calm, and alert much of the time. Here are four steps to help you attain (and sustain) the correct biochemical, physical, and psychological conditions:

1. Achieve Optimum Brain Nutrition.
A good diet and the right supplements provide you with the necessary building blocks for brain cells and neuro-transmitters, which are the mood, mind, and memory molecules. You will also be able to balance your blood sugar, which acts as brain and body fuel. This helps you to

break your dependency on substances that interfere with normal brain chemistry and deplete your energy.

It is vitally important to eat well in order to restore and maintain your brain function and remain substance abuse free. Here you will find a summary of good eating habits – the Healthy Brain Diet. You don't have to be in recovery to eat this way: It's the way we were meant to eat. This diet supports your brain function, energy, immunity, weight balance, and overall good health.

2. The Healthy Brain Diet

- Eat whole foods and fresh foods, organic whenever possible; avoid processed foods.

- Eat three servings a day of top-quality protein foods – fish, poultry, lean meat (free range), egg, soy, or combinations of beans, lentils, and grain

- Choose complex carbohydrates such as whole grains, vegetables, and most fruits, and avoid sugar and refined foods.

- Eat fish three times a week, or take fish-oil supplements.

- Drink at least a quart of water, if not two, day, either pure or in diluted juices and herbal or fruit teas.

- Minimize your intake of tea, coffee, and soft drinks.

- Eat lots of antioxidant-rich fruits and vegetables – at least five servings a day.

3. Get "fine-tuned" with natural supplements.

The reality of day-to-day life is that you will likely become stressed out or otherwise unbalanced. You will learn how to use natural substances to help bring yourself back into balance.

4. Think positively.

Chemistry isn't the whole story when it comes to feeling great. It's also about how we think. Ironically, while fear and anxiety seem to come easily, we often have to work harder to achieve happiness. Fortunately, you can replace negative patterns with a more positive and uplifting frame of mind – and there are specific methods to achieve this.

5. Adopt a mind- & mood-healthy lifestyle.

There are many ways to improve how you feel, specific lifestyle changes in the form of physical, mental, emotional, and spiritual exercises.

Chapter 7
Stimulants

You may want to seriously look at your relationship with stimulants. Keep a daily diary for three days or so, noting how much and when you consume: coffee, tea, chocolate, sugar, cigarettes or alcohol (both a stimulant and a relaxant). And indicate how intensely you crave them.

I find that my coffee-craving and alcoholic patients are often hypoglycemic and may also suffer from poor adrenal or thyroid function. The solution is a good medical evaluation, with treatment as necessary, including improved diet, exercise, and specific supplements. When these people reduce their dependence on caffeine, they are happily surprised to find that their overall energy level rises.

To get an idea of how depleted your energy might be and how dependent you are on energy stimulants, check yourself out in the following questionnaire:

* Do you have trouble getting up in the morning?

* Do you rely on a cup of coffee to get going in the morning?

* Do you feel tired all the time?

* Do you often feel foggy, fuzzy, or dull?

* Do you have trouble concentrating?

* Do you use sugar, caffeine (tea, coffee, caffeinated soft drinks), or cigarettes as a pick-me-up throughout the day?

- Do your moods seem to go up and down for no apparent reason?

- Are your mood swings often relieved by food, especially sweets?

- Do you have trouble falling asleep or staying asleep?

- Do you have headaches or shaky feelings that are relieved by sugar, caffeine, or cigarettes?

- Are you addicted to coffee, caffeinated soft drinks, energy drinks, or cigarettes?

- Do you find yourself constantly in crisis?

- Are you drawn to thrills, danger, and drama in your life?

If you had any "yes" answers, you are showing signs of depleted energy and may even be overly dependent on stimulants to keep you going. It is affecting your mental and physical health. Fortunately, you can get off them with the right diet, supplements, and lifestyle.

Breaking Free
Now let's look at stimulants in action – how they can addict you, and how to break free.

Jonathan, a 32-year old sales agent, had been a cocaine addict for several years. He explained how "after years of depression and no motivation, discovering cocaine actually made me feel normal for the first time in my life!" He also drank too much, and had some other extreme behaviors. He had destroyed his marriage through compulsive casual sex with other women and was heavily in debt from excessive gambling. He raised his brain's 'feel-good' chemicals with both cocaine and the adrenaline rush of thrill-seeking, risky behavior. The problem? He was requiring increasing amounts of everything just to stay even, while his life was falling apart around him.

The solution?

Here are Jonathan's own words:

"Fortunately, with the support of Gamblers Anonymous and Cocaine Anonymous, I was able to pull myself out of this mess, and recover some self- esteem. I started taking some vitamins that helped with my energy and cravings. I finally found the job I'm in – it's been three years now – and I've been clean the whole time. No drugs, alcohol, gambling, or chasing after women. I realized that those "bored" feelings were depression, and the coke and alcohol made me feel normal, at least briefly. I've been helped enormously by my vitamins, the 12-Step programs, eating right, and exercising regularly.

"I don't even drink coffee or use sugar – I found that they were as addictive as drugs, and would give me the same pattern of highs and lows. My ADD (attention deficit disorder) is under control, too. I can concentrate, remember things, and keep my desk and my life organized for the first time in my life. It's been a hard road but I can honestly say, I have never felt better. Let me tell you, drugs just aren't worth it. I've been there and back, and I know."

What was Jonathan's problem? Moral weakness? Poor upbringing? Bad luck? Knowing the source of the problem helps us to find the solution. As it turned out, Jonathan was suffering from what researcher, Dr. Kenneth Blum, has termed *"Reward Deficiency Syndrome,"* or "RDS." People with RDS are born with a tendency toward low moods and have difficulty feeling "normal."

While extreme, Jonathan's out-of-control addiction to cocaine, gambling, alcohol, fast living, and high-risk behavior helps us to understand the full range of the problem. He had a biological tendency toward RDS, and once he started using, couldn't stop. Even in "normal" people, repeated use of certain substances can lead to addiction, as can stress itself.

Treatment Issues

Jonathan's only escape was to gradually stop using the substances. By taking natural supplements, he was able to restore chemical balance, and end his cravings. His reward deficiency was due to low dopamine.

With adequate neurotransmitter building blocks, such as D,L-phenylalanine (DLPA), L-glutamine, and tyrosine, 500 mg of each 3 times daily, and 5-HTP, 200 mg daily, his mood became normal, without the depression and anxiety that he had always plagued him.

Jonathan began taking the Brain Recovery AM & PM capsules that contain not only most of these ingredients, but also blood- sugar balancing and liver detoxifying nutrients, supplied in 2 convenient bottles. Initially, he needed extra 5-HTP (100–200 mg more than the 100 mg contained in the PM bottle) and extra doses of the stimulating amino acids, DLPA and tyrosine, as found in my FOCUS formula, 2–4 capsules daily.

Jonathan likely also benefited from the amino acid, N-acetyl-cysteine (NAC), which is contained in the formula. Research shows that NAC is a powerful treatment for addiction and other brain issues, like depression, gambling, and even Alzheimer's Disease. NAC is a precursor to the master antioxidant, glutathione, which is made in the liver and is required to counter the brain inflammation that is so much a part of all these conditions. This topic is beyond the scope of this book, but a promising thesis and approach to treatment.

You may wonder how he could overcome a biological, and most likely genetic problem with such low-tech medicine. Here's the answer:

We are not simply victims of our genetic make-up. Genetics give only the predisposition to a condition. Its actual manifestation, or *expression*, can be influenced and changed by diet, supplements and lifestyle.

Jonathan was thus able to take measures, as can you, to control how these genes were expressed; that is, how they actually affected him. By understanding our propensities, we can take the appropriate preventive steps. Or do good remedial work if we have already been affected.

This model applies to the use of caffeine, sugar, chocolate, and tobacco, as well. Each has its own way of stimulating the reward system, but the end result is the same. They all lead to a rise in blood sugar and dopamine, and the brain becomes addicted to them. We become slaves to the dopamine rush!

Treatment Options

Of course I also see my share of patients who are already in various stages of recovery from alcohol, cocaine, marijuana, opiates, etc. But in all cases, the treatment is similar, and not very complicated, despite all the scientific jargon here.

The good news is, you don't have to 'power through' the recovery process. There are ways to cut the cravings to a minimum, by taking the right supplements. As in Margo's case (see below), I may not even have to address the problem head on. I learned this early in my career of nutritional psychiatry, and rather by accident.

Stimulants – You Don't Need Them

While stimulants can create energy in the short run, the long-term effect is always bad. The same is true for stress. So the first step to beating stress and fatigue is to cut out, or cut down on, stimulants. That means, as we've noted, coffee (including decaf), tea, chocolate, sugar and refined foods, cigarettes, cola drinks and alcohol.

By eating slow-releasing carbohydrates and taking energy nutrients as supplements, you can minimize withdrawal symptoms, which usually last no more that four days. Then try the substance again, and notice what happens with your first tea, coffee, hit of sugar, or chocolate.

You'll experience what Dr. Hans Selye, father of the general adaptation syndrome and stress response, called the *initial response or Phase 1* – in other words, a true response to these powerful chemicals: pounding head, hyperactive mind, fast heartbeat and insomnia, followed by extreme drowsiness.

Keep on the stimulants and you will *adapt – that's Phase 2*. Keep doing this long enough and eventually you hit *exhaustion – Phase 3*. This happens to everybody, the only variable being how long takes you to get to the "exhaustion" phase.

Recovery from stimulants is not only possible, it's usually very rapid. With nutritional support, most people have substantially more energy and ability to cope with stress within thirty days of quitting stimulants. So hang in there!

Here are some tips to help you get started.

- Identify the stimulants you are addicted to.

- Follow the Healthy Brain Diet (page 89)

- Eat a hypoglycemic diet: i.e. small, frequent meals

- Find which substitutes you like the most, and avoid or considerably reduce your intake of stimulants until they are no longer a daily requirement.

- Notice your patterns of stressful response and replace them with a more positive one

- Integrate exercise into your life

- Take the recommended supplements or simply take Brain Recovery AM & PM Formula which you may have to augment at first with additional amino acids.

Coffee and Caffeine

It takes four days on average to break the coffee habit, longer if you're a slow metabolizer and also majorly addicted. During this time you may experience headaches and drowsiness. These are a strong reminder of how bad coffee really is for you. Decaffeinated coffee contains some caffeine, and is just a little better. A delicious natural coffee alternative is grain-based Teeccino, available at many health food stores and by mail-order. When brewed, it even tastes like the real thing.

Is Tea OK?

Try a lower caffeine tea, or green tea, and then move on to caffeine-free herbal teas. Regular green tea isn't caffeine free, but contains much less caffeine than regular tea and has other health benefits. It's also a good appetite suppressant. There's L-theanine, to enhance brain alpha states, making you calm and alert at the same time. You can drink 2–3 cups max daily. Or drink it decaf, with all the same healthy ingredients, like antioxidants that protect against heart disease and cancer, according to Harvard research.

What About Chocolate?

Among other ingredients, chocolate contains phenethylamine (PEA), a pleasurable brain stimulant related to phenylalanine, making chocolate "the love drug." Chocolate also contains magnesium, fat and sugar. There is usually one of these ingredients that is your nemesis. If you can't figure out which it is, these supplements cover all four:

- **D,L-Phenylalanine**: 500–1,000 mg, 2–3 times daily
- **Magnesium**: 200–300 mg twice daily
- **Fat**: flax or hemp oil, 1 tablespoon twice daily
- **Sugar**: see hypoglycemic diet and supplement plan

Energy Drinks

Are you hooked on energy drinks? Gotta have that Red Bull or Monster? Well, they are quite depleting and negatively impact your health. We have a solution. You can get a more natural and sustained boost from taking my FOCUS formula, along with some other products. My products are all modular and do well together, so no worries about "mixing and matching" them. There is more information, too, in my ebook, *Reclaim Your Brain*. (For your free copy, visit: http://cassmd.com/reclaimsignup.)

Suggested Formulas:
You can start with FOCUS, then add in Energy Boost and Super EPA. For a total approach, add the Brain Recovery AM & PM Formula.

- **FOCUS for brain energy, focus, and concentration:** 2 caps 1–2 times daily

- **Energy Boost for the adrenal glands:** 2 caps 1–2 times daily

- **Super EPA:** 1 capsule twice daily

- **Brain Recovery AM & PM formula:** 5–7 capsules of each once daily: AM with breakfast and PM with dinner.

Chapter 8
Alcohol

Here is a story that may seem familiar – if not for you, then for someone you know. Your own story may be more about sugar or caffeine, or any substance with which you have this relationship. Or you may have no addictions at all. Nonetheless, the information I'm about to give you applies to anyone with a brain, since that is where the action is! If you've ever wondered what made you tick, I can provide some answers.

Margo, a 35-year-old flight attendant, consulted me for a "tune-up." She noticed that she was more tired and less able to adapt to time zone changes than in the past. When I asked her to describe her diet, she was quick to plead, "Don't make me give up my drink with dinner!"

I didn't even say the "A" word, for "alcoholic." Who am I to judge, or give her a pejorative label for which she would resent me, or become defensive? That is, if she did decide to stop, it would be by choice, and with no guilt or suffering, either, and without needing to use white-knuckling willpower. Believe it or not, with the right nutrients, cravings can be stopped quickly and often painlessly, as you will see!

It was Margo's attachment to her drink that was the clue to how dependent she was on it. If alcohol had held no emotional charge for her she wouldn't have even thought of mentioning it. *We're not talking about the one drink a day. We're talking about the attitude.* Substitute any other addiction and you'll see what we mean: the late-afternoon candy bar, the eagerly anticipated cigarette break or one's morning coffee.

When people like Margo have problems with a substance, it's usually not that they are weak-willed or have an "addictive personality." They simply have an underlying chemical imbalance that is depleting their energy and peace of mind and they don't even know it. As you'll see, it's your brain chemistry that "makes you do it."

Now you may protest, "but I just like my morning coffee...or 'my after-work beer with my friends...' or 'my glass of wine with dinner...I could give it up any time." And often these habits appear to be just tension relievers, pick-me-ups, or one of the normal pleasures of life. But are they? Generally not, and I will tell you why. You can then apply this to your own life, and see what fits.

Whether it's sugar, caffeine, alcohol, soft drinks or tobacco, your dependence on them undermines your health. I seldom tell my patients that they "have to" stop or even reduce these addictive substances – as if knowing that they 'should' would make a difference! And we have better ways.

Curbing Alcohol Cravings with Amino Acids

Research shows that we can successfully treat addiction with the use of specific amino acids. These include materials that are made into our brain chemical messengers, the *neurotransmitters* – serotonin, dopamine, norepinephrine, endorphins, and GABA.

When neurotransmitters precursors were given to alcoholic individuals, they experienced the following:

- Fewer cravings for alcohol

- A reduced incidence of stress

- An increased likelihood of recovery

- Reduction in relapse rates

How many programs can boast that record? And again, willpower has nothing to do with it. In fact, one experiment created alcoholic rats, who were found to prefer alcohol to water. Once they were given the right mix of nutrients, however, their alcoholism resolved. No willpower needed!

Margo began a vitamin program that included 500–1000 mg of the amino acid L-glutamine under her tongue, at the times when she would usually consider a drink. Sure enough, she noticed that she no longer was craving her glass of wine. Before long, she could barely even remember how important it had been to her. This convenient forgetting is an interesting phenomenon that I have seen over and over again.

In addition to taking the supplements I prescribed, Margo also completed my detox plan (see page 40) and learned a great deal about herself. After being off of sugar for a week, when Margo added sugar to her herbal tea, she became wired. And about an hour later, Margo reported that she felt very sleepy.

It was clear to me that she was still quite burned out at that stage and her adrenals had little reserve, giving her that exaggerated response. These reactions had been occurring all along but had been "masked" by her long-term sugar habit. That's why it's a good idea to stop potential problem foods and then watch your response when they are slowly reintroduced, one at a time.

Margo didn't even want to test herself on alcohol. Had she not been taking supplements, I would also have been concerned about her going off the wagon. As it turned out, there was no problem here. Her need for a daily drink (or more) of wine ended quite easily. As her nutritional status improved with a good diet, multi-vitamins and amino acids, she "forgot'" her habit. The last opened bottle of wine actually sat in the refrigerator until her roommate finally used it for cooking!

A Brain in Balance

The secret is that once you are on a well-balanced and nutritious diet and taking the right supplements, the cravings disappear. That's because they are symptoms of an imbalance that, once corrected, frees you of the compulsion. You are then able to choose a drink with dinner or a cookie for dessert (and not a whole box of them, a sign of sugar addiction). Or not. There is no inner conflict involved here. You're free! Please don't take this as license to drink if you are genetically predisposed to alcoholism, even when protected by supplements, since slips happen.

When diet alone doesn't work, research shows we can successfully treat addiction and cravings with the use of specific amino acids. These include the precursors (building blocks) of the neurotransmitters serotonin, dopamine, glutamine, and GABA (gamma-amino-butyric acid, which is both a neurotransmitter and an amino acid)

If you have cravings for fast food, doughnuts and high-sugar foods, coffee, tea, soft drinks, chocolate, alcohol or any other substance, we have a simple answer for you – read on.

Here's another great story about alcohol use.

Bruce, a 35-year-old realtor with a high pressure, competitive job came to see me for anxiety, depression, and low energy. His intake questionnaire revealed that he drank a six-pack of beer every two days or so. Ignoring that specific issue, we began several sessions of counseling, including stress reduction techniques such as meditation.

I also prescribed a series of supplements to address his physiological imbalances, including a high potency multivitamin-mineral formula with high B vitamin content, chromium 200 mcg twice daily (for blood sugar balance), tyrosine 500–1000 mg twice daily for energy, and glutamine, 500 mg three times a day, for low mood and substance cravings. For his convenience, I later shifted him over to the Brain Recovery capsules.

When I asked two months later about his beer drinking, he first gave me a blank look, then lit up and exclaimed, "Funny you should ask. I just noticed a six-pack that had been sitting in the refrigerator for weeks, untouched, and kind of wondered why I hadn't been drinking." With Bruce, as with Margo, not only do the habits disappear, but so does the feeling-state and memory of their even having been there.

"Who, me? I don't remember doing that!"

When someone corrects an emotional issue, or even a physical symptom, there is often a kind of amnesia about it. It is as if the "normal" person they have become no longer has the space to carry around the formerly unbalanced self in their head. They no longer live in the damage of the past, and old behaviors and relationships are replaced with healthier ones.

Contrary to what some psychotherapists might say (and may be true in certain cases), I don't classify this response as "pathological denial." Rather, it is a tribute to the ability of the human being to grow beyond adversity and to flower. You leave your old self behind, like a butterfly releasing its cocoon and its prior existence as a caterpillar. The old life is history.

Alcohol: It's Just One Drink!

It is all too easy to overindulge in alcohol because of its role in social interaction. Start by limiting the times you have alcohol, such as your lunchtime drink. You'll certainly work better in the afternoon. Ideally, cut it out completely for at least the first two weeks. If you find this hard to do, take a close look at your drinking habits, and, if necessary, seek professional help. Alcoholics Anonymous is a great resource, as well, but often not sufficient since it doesn't address the physical underpinnings.

There is a great deal of self-deception that goes on in the name of "just social drinking." Some signs that you have a drinking problem:

• Your friends or spouse tells you that you drink too much.

- You have been arrested for drinking while driving (no, it's not "just those dumb cops!").

- You look forward to dinner because it's preceded by a martini and accompanied by a bottle of wine.

- Revisit the quiz in chapter 4.

Be especially concerned if alcoholism runs in your family. Above all remember: excessive drinking is a reflection of a brain imbalance, not a crime, but can turn into one if you don't do something about quitting.

Note: The program for alcohol detox is similar to both the stimulant withdrawal and the tranquilizer protocol; so, if this is you, please look at both.

Chapter 9
Sugar

Refined sugar adds calories and has no food value. What's more, high-sugar foods like soft drinks, doughnuts and candy lead to a mood roller coaster called the "sugar blues." First these foods cause a rapid rise in blood sugar (glucose), requiring your body to secrete more insulin to cope with it. The insulin then removes this excess sugar from the blood and stores it as fat and glycogen. This causes your blood sugar levels to drop and making you feel weak, light-headed and even cranky.

What about sugar substitutes? Diet drinks contain the artificial sweetener aspartame (brand names Nutra-Sweet, Equal), which can be toxically over-stimulating to the brain. I've seen patients who thought they were going crazy with jitters, insomnia and disordered thinking. Instead, they magically recovered when they stopped drinking diet sodas! Ironically, too, while touted as a diet product, these drinks can actually cause weight gain. When consumed with carbohydrates, aspartame inhibits the production of a brain chemical that signals fullness. You can find many articles on line about the dangers of aspartame, including this one on Livestrong.com.

To get over an aspartame addiction, try the amino acid D,L phenylalanine, a relative of tyrosine.

Splenda®, the trade name for sucralose, produced by chlorinating sugar (sucrose), is no better. Do you really want to ingest chlorine, a toxic halogen that, cells from absorbing and utilizing iodine, a mineral that is essential for thyroid function and even cancer prevention. There have been no long-term human studies on Splenda®'s use and no independent monitoring of health effects. However, animal studies show it to be dangerous in many ways.

Eliminating sugar, artificially sweetened and caffeine-containing soft drinks will move you strongly in the right direction.

To take care of those other cravings, you can substitute a 2-ounce pack of raw (and preferably unsalted) nuts for your afternoon candy bar and you won't get sugar withdrawal. In fact, you'll probably experience quite the opposite. You'll notice the difference in your energy levels right away. Most nuts are excellent sources of healthy fats. Almonds, cashews, and walnuts are particularly good sources of protein as well.

If you really like your sweets, try xylitol, an excellent sugar substitute that has health benefits as well: it helps to prevent tooth decay by preventing the growth of bacteria in the mouth. Another good choice is stevia, a sweet herbal extract that may even help lower blood sugar. Stevia is easily found at health food stores in both liquid and powdered form. It works best in drinks. It doesn't work as well in baking because heating changes the flavor.

The addition of complex carbohydrates, including more high-fiber foods, will go a long way toward allaying your sugar cravings. Add some protein and a dose of chromium (200 mcg), and you are far less likely to go on a sugar binge.

For both sugar and alcohol cravings, balance your sugar and add 500 mg of glutamine twice daily, and as needed under the tongue. This little step has miraculously turned around a number of my heavy-drinking patients relatively painlessly.

Hint for Handling Cravings

Take 1 or 2 500 mg capsules of L-glutamine, open, and pour the powdered contents under your tongue. It is absorbed quickly, and gives a pick-up similar to that of your longed-for stimulant, including alcohol. You can also take a 500 mg capsule several times a day, between meals, to prevent cravings.

A reader named Lucy sent me the following unsolicited e-mail, two months after we met at a presentation that I'd given on natural approaches to addiction. I suggested that she try glutamine for her alcohol addiction.

"I've had three wonderfully clean weeks since you gave me the name of the "magical" powder. It didn't seem possible – but it was immediate. For me it was a miracle (do you also walk on water?!).

In addition: I've lost 10 lbs. I lost my daily morning cough. My complexion is so much clearer I have four to six more hours of daily LIFE. Best of all, I feel like a different person, a new personality.

So I thank you very much...my life is changed. I stand still and study my body to see why I don't crave a drink...is it in my brain?

Why doesn't AA and the CDC and all the doctors know about this magic over-the-counter item?" — Lucy

Lucy's weight loss was a 'side benefit,' since glutamine reduces carb cravings by raising brain blood sugar. It also reduces food allergies by healing the lining of the gastrointestinal tract, which is often inflamed in alcoholics. This would also help her absorb her nutrients better. Her clearer complexion was likely also due to glutamine's positive effect of helping absorb nutrients and promote detoxification. I prescribe it frequently to recovering alcoholics for that reason.

Add 500 mg of D,L-phenylalanine or tyrosine two to three times a day, and your energy will be high and stay that way, with no more cravings! Both are found in Dr. Cass' FOCUS Formula.

Chapter 10
Carbohydrates

As you can see, it's not only alcohol and drugs that are addictive. Food addiction, and carbohydrates in particular, is a major issue for many people, especially women, as we see in Kim's case.

On the surface, her situation was not unusual. A successful 38-year-old professional, Kim was a single working mother of two energetic teenagers, and found herself with an ever- growing list of unfinished tasks.

Exhausted and near burnout, she felt stretched emotionally, financially, and professionally. She would "collapse into bed in a heap" at night and fall asleep easily. However, she would often awaken at 3 or 4 a.m., her heart pounding, her mind racing, and unable to fall back to sleep until just before the alarm rang at 6:30. It didn't matter what time she went to bed, either.

Kim's diet was fast food, doughnuts and coffee, consumed on the run. She suffered from frequent headaches, heart palpitations, and at times, shakiness. Her symptoms pointed to hypoglycemia or low blood sugar, which can appear in many forms: depression, irritability, anxiety, panic attacks, fatigue, "brain fog," headaches (including migraines), insomnia, muscular weakness, and tremors. All of these symptoms may be relieved by food, as in her case, the more sugary the better. So she ended up craving sweets, coffee, alcohol, or drugs; in fact, many addictions are related to hypoglycemia.

When Kim ate high glycemic foods, such as dough-nuts and candy, or drank coffee, her blood sugar levels rose rapidly. This led to a large, quick release of insulin, which then removed the sugar from circulation, storing it as fat and glycogen. This caused her blood sugar level to drop over the next one to two hours, making Kim feel weak, lightheaded, and even cranky. When this cycle repeated itself enough, the overtaxed adrenal glands became exhausted – and so did she.

Why did she continue to overindulge in pasta, cookies, chips, candies, ice cream, and donuts, while ignoring what she know to be true about them? What was so irresistible about them? Her brain (and good judgment) had been hijacked!

The Solution

To support Kim's adrenals and balance her blood sugar, I recommended the following:

First, I prescribed dietary changes, including cut-ting out refined carbohydrates, such as sugar and white flour, plus no coffee or alcohol. I also recommended small, frequent meals containing protein and complex carbo-hydrates, which have a low glycemic index (low-GI). This index measures how quickly a specific food is turned into glucose, or blood sugar, which in turn stimulates the pancreas to release insulin.

The result? Vegetables and whole grains allowed for more stable blood-glucose levels, which increased her energy and her ability to handle stress. The complex carbohydrates also helped raise her serotonin levels, which both calmed her down and lifted her mood. Serotonin is sensitive to shifts in female hormones, too, explaining the sugar cravings that often accompany PMS. That's why I recommend avoiding sugar especially during PMS, and adding in a serotonin enhancer like 5-HTP.

Supplements

I prescribed a daily nutritional supplement regimen for Kim. This included: A high potency multi-vitamin-mineral with meals for basic support, also containing adequate doses of nutrients that to help balance blood sugar and support the adrenals: B vitamins, chromium, vanadium, magnesium, manganese, potassium, zinc, pantothenic acid (Vitamin B5), 2 g and vitamin C, 2,000 mg.

In the morning, two of my Energy Boost capsules containing adaptogenic herbs helped restore and support her overworked adrenal glands, and an extra two with lunch to prevent her afternoon slump.

She also needed 5-HTP to raise her serotonin levels: 100 mg in the morning and 200 mg at bedtime (starting at 100 then increased). It helped balance blood sugar, lower anxiety, raise her mood, enhance sleep, and stop her carb cravings. Not bad for one single amino acid!

For cravings, I recommended my favorite sugar balancer: glutamine 500 mg under the tongue, and in capsules, 2–3 times daily.

Exercise

Kim began to exercise regularly, which allowed her to burn fats, maintain blood sugar levels, relieve anxiety, and up her mood. Research proves that regular exercise can actually reduce the amount of adrenal hormones the body releases in response to stress. In addition, it raises the level of the mood-elevating hormones, or endorphins, in the brain. You know, a runner's high!

Results

Kim's new habits had a marked effect on stabilizing her moods. Her physical symptoms cleared, too. There were no more early morning awakenings, no more headaches, and no more fatigue. The stresses of life as a busy mother and office worker continued, but she no longer fell victim to her inner chemistry. She now had an internal buffer against stress – functioning adrenal glands and a smoother supply of blood sugar to her body, particularly to her brain.

She graduated to taking my Brain Recovery AM & PM capsules containing the supplements mentioned above, with a side of Energy Boost, two every morning with a early afternoon booster if needed, during periods when she felt more tired or stressed.

The predisposition to hypoglycemia runs in families, so if you have a family history of diabetes, pre-diabetes, or hypoglycemia, you need to be more attentive to stress, diet, and nutritional supplements.

Relaxation techniques are useful, too, and once balance is restored, you may want some psychotherapy to help reveal and deal with the underlying psychodynamics. Otherwise you're running a constant "stress program" in the background messing up your brain/computer. Therapy reboots your computer, eliminating old, bad programs so you can live life in the present as you were meant to, without all the old baggage.

Chapter 11
Nicotine

Nicotine can be as addictive as heroin, which makes quitting smoking difficult. Even in small doses, nicotine produces a substantial effect. It can give you a lift, cut your appetite, and, at tense times, can relax you. All of these effects are due to nicotine's action on adrenal hormones, blood sugar and brain chemicals.

If you quite cold turkey, you'll likely feel irritable, agitated, hungry, and desperate for a smoke. The low blood sugar can leave you feeling nauseous, flu-ish, moody, and craving sweets. However, by following the Basic Detox Diet (Chap 20) and the Brain Recovery Prescription (Chap 23), the craving for cigarettes will diminish as you stabilize your blood sugar and hormone levels.

So, before you even begin to try to quit cigarettes, *I recommend following these diet and supplement guidelines for a month or so*, until you no longer consume any other stimulants, such as tea, coffee, chocolate, or sugar. Instead you'll be eating small, frequent meals, with an emphasis on foods containing slow-releasing carbohydrates combined with foods rich in protein.

You are likely addicted to smoking at particular times, such as when you're tired, hungry or upset, on waking, with a drink after a meal, or after sex. Note what these cues are, and separate them from smoking, one by one. You will be left with 'just smoking.'

Then reduce your nicotine load gradually, switching to brands that contain less nicotine until down to no more than 2 mg per cigarette (or the equivalent in chewing tobacco or e-cigarettes). At this point you can quit, though many will temporarily turn to nicotine gum. However, I have discovered a promising new alternative, with a faster onset and greater bioavailability than the gum. Taken in a "step down" program in decreasing doses over 90 days – 3, 2, 1, and 0 mg – it is a nicotine-infused *dental stick* (i.e. toothpick). It has some other advantages too, such as offering longer-lasting oral gratification, since people tend to keep them in their mouths longer.

Start the **Basic Detox Diet** and begin exercising daily to enhance endorphins. If you're tired, add in an adrenal support formula like **Energy Boost.**

Nicotine depletes a variety of neurotransmitters, so start with the list below along with a high potency multi, such as my **Twice Daily Better Balance Multi**, or simply take my **Brain Recovery AM&PM** which covers them all and more (details in Chapter 23). Then, if needed, you can add these supplements twice daily, since they are in higher doses than in Brain Recovery.

- **Vitamin C** 1,000 mg or more, to bowel tolerance, i.e., until you feel gassy or have loose stools, then back down by one capsule or so.

- **Chromium** 100 mcg–200 mcg to balance blood sugar.

- **Tyrosine** 500–1,000 mg twice daily or Dr. Cass' FOCUS formula, 2 capsules twice daily.

- **Niacin** 500–2,000 mg; or non-flush niacin, same dose.

You may experience a flushing sensation when first taking niacin, 15 to 30 minutes after taking it, and lasting for about 15 minutes. It helps to take it with a meal, though over time, the flush response will stop occurring, anyway.

Or instead, use either non-flush form: inositol hexanicotinate (niacinate) or niacinamide

- **Calcium** (about 600 mg) and **Magnesium** (about 600 mg) daily are alkaline minerals and help to neutralize excess the acidity that adds to the craving. For cravings, eat fruit instead of having a smoke. This will raise a low blood sugar level, which is often the trigger. There are 600 mg of magnesium in the Brain Recovery AM & PM program capsules.

- **5-hydroxytryptophan** (5-HTP) 100–300 mg daily, in divided doses with greater dose 1 hour before bed, since serotonin levels rise at night and promote sleep. Or take its relative, trytophan, 1000–3,000 mg, which needs some carb to help it get across the blood-brain barrier. Nicotine withdrawal tends to lower serotonin levels, leaving you depressed and irritable.

- **Glutamine** 500–1,000 mg as needed for cravings, under the tongue for quicker action, to balance blood sugar, and produce a calming effect since it converts to GABA

In addition to Brain Recovery AM&PM, you'll need:

- **Brain Cell Support Plus** 1–2 capsules twice daily to build and protect brain cells. It also provides citicoline, a precursor to the memory neurotransmitter acetylcholine, which is used up in smoking.

- **Omega-3 fatty acids** 1,000 mg twice daily

For further details see Section 3.

Chapter 12
Marijuana/Cannabis

Despite assertions to the contrary by many, I have seen marijuana be one of those "I'm not addicted, I can quit when I want to," substances – where the people involved don't know they're addicted till they try to stop and find out how difficult it is. Or they finally do clean up and find they have a clearer mind, are functioning much better than when they were smoking regularly.

The immediate effects of smoking cannabis are feeling high and a little drowsy, though there are some cultivars that are more stimulating. Research shows that the brain responds to cannabis by releasing the feel-good neurotransmitter, dopamine.

Cannabis's effects on judgment, coordination, and short-term memory make it a bad idea to drive, to operate heavy machinery, or to try to learn anything new while under its influence. This is due to the high concentration of cannabis receptors in both the hippocampus, the part of the brain that controls memory, and the cerebellum, the part of the brain that governs motor coordination. Moreover, these effects may actually last longer than those of alcohol.

Here's the experience of Gene, a forty-five-year-old, married physical therapist:

I'd only smoke a hit or two every other day, but I had been doing this for years. I finally stopped smoking marijuana completely eight months ago and I feel a lot better. My workouts have improved, and my overall energy level is up. When I smoked, I would feel relaxed at first, but after an hour or so, my mood would dip. I'd get cranky and want another hit. The next one wouldn't do it, though, so I gave up trying. The moodiness was probably due to a low blood-sugar reaction – you know, "the munchies." Then, I'd eat, so I put on too much weight.

I finally decided I'd had enough of it all, and just quit. I became really irritable. Not only was I craving a smoke, but I had to handle all kinds of emotional issues that were coming up, things I hadn't ever dealt with. Fortunately, I had some aromatherapy and herbal products that really helped cut the cravings and lift my mood.

Eventually, after about six to eight weeks, my moods evened out. Now, if I find myself wanting a joint to relax, I take a whiff of my aromatherapy oil or a dose of kava. Overall, I'm glad to be over the whole thing. Life feels more real to me now. My wife likes me better now, too. She says I'm more emotionally available, more stable, and nicer to be with!

In my own observation, young people who smoke their way through high school and continue through young adulthood are more likely to have problems. They are often less able to cope with the challenges of everyday life or to plan appropriately for their futures. Their emotional development seems blunted: the marijuana fog may have prevented them from fully experiencing a complete range of emotions and relationships. Stoned on the hero's journey, they miss the passages necessary for growing up and accepting their place in the adult world.

I am not addressing medical marijuana here. I discussed it in detail in Natural Highs. However, recreational use, and overuse, is a different issue, since despite what many may protest, it is addictive, with tolerance and withdrawal. And, as mentioned, it's not a good idea for young people.

To restore overall brain and neurotransmitter balance, see Section 3.

Specific to marijuana are the following:
Eat high density, high-fat and high protein food, organic butter, eggs, and beans which help you restart making your own natural *anandamide* the feel-good neurotransmitter that is disrupted by pot use.
Omega 3 fatty acids 2000 mg twice daily
Borage oil 2000 mg twice daily, an anandamide precursor

To enhance acetylcholine production, disrupted by marijuana use, and repair the cell membrane, add:
Phospholipids such as citicoline and phosphatidyl serine contained in Brain Cell Support, 1-2 capsules twice daily
  - or lecithin granules 1000-2000 mg twice daily

Chapter 13

Opiates: Heroin, Codeine, and Painkillers

The opiates such as oxycontin, vicodin, meperidine (Demerol), and heroin are in the family of drugs that cause a feeling of great calm and pleasure, an escape from it all. All highly addictive, they are the part of current addiction epidemic. They use up your dopamine and endorphins, leading to a painful withdrawal. Symptoms include anxiety, muscle tension, diarrhea, stomach pains, flu-like symptoms and more. While most pronounced in the first 24 hours, the symptoms can go on for a month or more.

Supplement list, taken twice daily:

- GABA, glutamine, taurine, glycine – 100 mg each or Dr. Cass' CALM Natural Mind 2 capsules

- NAC 500 mg

- Niacinamide 500 mg

- 5-HTP 100 mg

- Magnesium 150 mg

- Vitamin C 1000 mg every hour (or to bowel tolerance)

- Or: Dr. Cass' Brain Recovery AM&PM Formula which includes all of the above, as a base and reinforce as needed (see section 3)

Chapter 14

Tranquilizers

If you take anti-anxiety drugs, you have lots of company. More than 4 million Americans take prescription benzo-diazepines such as Valium or Xanax every day, often for years. Two-thirds of all prescriptions for benzodiazepine are written by family practitioners, and the remainder by psychiatrists. Highly addictive, they are also responsible for a major portion of accidents, many serious and even fatal. Benzodiazepines happen to be one of the largest classes of abused drugs, as well.

Minimizing Withdrawal Symptoms with Natural Remedies

Coming off benzodiazepines has its own hazards, and must be done under medical supervision. Abruptly withdrawing from high doses can lead to seizures and even death.

My patient Marcy had been hooked on Valium, and finally took herself off it, cold turkey. Not a good idea. She had a many of the usual withdrawal symptoms: insomnia, anxiety, irritability, sweating, blurred vision, diarrhea, tremors, mental impairment and headaches.

Had she known better, she would have gone on a gradual program of withdrawal coupled with natural remedies such as theanine, GABA, and valerian, as found in CALM Natural Mind, and Nightly CALM, both of which can ease and shorten the transition phase.

The ideal withdrawal program has to be tailored to the unique circumstances – the amount of the drug taken, length of use, and your unique physiology. It takes months to get off these drugs completely, and professional support and guidance are essential.

As mentioned, the herb, valerian, is also a great help in the process of withdrawal. A GABA enhancer, it will have similar actions to the drug, but is much gentler and doesn't have the same addictive potential. The same is true for GABA and theanine. You gradually reduce the tranquilizer dose while increasing that of the supplements. Experiment with each, and see which one works best for you. They each have their own actions and "feel," so the choice depends on how well they're doing the job.

A word of caution – since benzodiazepines, GABA, theanine, and valerian all enhance GABA, the combination of the herbs with tranquilizer drugs can make the drugs' effects more potent.

For this reason, valerian, as well as the amino acids theanine and GABA, should be viewed in the same way as any medicine, and taken in carefully scheduled doses as part of the medically supervised withdrawal program.

To sum up, here are some practical steps you can take to break addiction to tranquilizers, and minimize symptoms of withdrawal:

- Do this only under the guidance of a physician.

- Deal with psychological issues with the guidance of a psychotherapist.

- Start with milk thistle (*Silymarin silibum*), a supportive herb for the liver, your detox factory, to speed up the break-down of these drugs in your body. Alpha lipoic acid is also an excellent liver support, even used intravenously for acute liver toxicity as occurs in acute mushroom poisoning. Both nutrients are found in my Brain Recovery AM&PM Formula.

- Gradually reduce the tranquilizer dose, under professional guidance, and replace it with valerian, theanine, glycine and/or taurine. Or take my CALM Natural Mind which contains all of these: 2 capsules as needed throughout the day, for maximum of 8 capsules per day. Space them at least 2 hours away from the medication, to avoid interaction since they have similar effects.

- When withdrawal symptoms are gone, along with the meds, reduce the supplement doses. Since they are not addictive and do not build tolerance, you don't have to be weaned off them later.

- Follow the Healthy Brain Diet guidelines

Chapter 15

SSRI Withdrawal

More and more information is coming to light about withdrawal problems from the Selective Serotonin Reuptake Inhibitors or SSRI antidepressants, such as fluoxetine (Prozac), Sertraline (Zoloft, Lustral), Paroxetine (Paxil), Citalopram (Celexa), and Escitalopram (Lexapro), to name the most popular. Even more difficult are the SNRI or serotonin-norepinephrine reuptake inhibitors, such as Venlafaxine (brand names: Effexor, Effexor XR). Experts assert that technically, none of these are addictive. However, there are definite issues of tolerance and withdrawal that must be addressed.

In his books, *Prozac Backlash*, and *The Antidepressant Solution*, Harvard psychiatrist Joseph Glenmullen begins by describing the serious long-term side effects associated with these serotonin-boosting medications. I have found the same in my own practice, where individuals consult me to help them wean off the meds.

They include neurological disorders, such as facial and whole-body tics ('tardive dyskinesia') that can indicate brain damage; sexual dysfunction in at least 60 percent of users; debilitating withdrawal symptoms, including visual hallucinations, electric shock-like sensations in the brain (brain zaps), dizziness, nausea, and anxiety; and a decrease of antidepressant effectiveness in about 35 percent of long-term users.

In addition, his research points to the direct link between these drugs, and suicide and violence. See also my Huffington Post blog on the subject (http://www.huffingtonpost.com/hyla-cass-md/is-it-drugs-not-guns-that_b_2393385.html)

There is research showing that the SSRIs also make you prone to weight gain, and, when taken by pregnant women, to birth defects in the fetus.

Unless you wean off any psychotropic (mind-altering) medication very slowly, you can go into withdrawal, euphemistically called "discontinuation syndrome" by the medical profession. Symptoms include bouts of overwhelming depression, 'brain zaps' (fortunately, often relieved by fish oil), insomnia, and fatigue.

It can even include life-threatening physical effects, psychosis, or violent outbursts. Sadly, many psychiatrists cavalierly minimize these problems.

The irony here is that research shows that for most users, the effects are largely placebo, but one with potentially serious side effects. (Fournier JC, DeRubeis RJ, et al. "Antidepressant drug effects and depression severity," *JAMA* 2010; 303(1):47-53.

Another problem is that they stop working after a while and either the dose needs to be increased, the product changed to a different one, or another one added. Why? The receptor sites downregulate or close down, and more serotonin is needed to have the same effect. But in fact, the drugs actually deplete serotonin. So you are chasing the elusive goal of keeping a healthy serotonin level unless you help Mother Nature by giving the brain the material it needs. (see p. 25)

Basic Weaning Protocol:

A good solution here is to add serotonin precursors, i.e., the amino acid 5-hydroxytryptophan (5-HTP) along with B vitamins especially B6, B12 and folate, or take a potent multivitamin that contains a good dose of them, such as my Two Daily Better Balance Multi, or Brain Recovery AM&PM. They both also contain methylfolate, a form of folic acid that can actually enter the cell more readily. This is especially useful for a significant per cent of the population, especially many of those suffering from depression due to a defect in this area.

Then reduce the medication by 10% every 7-14 days, unless or until there are symptoms of withdrawal, then return to the last comfortable dose and wait a longer interval. Toward the end, you may have to make the reductions even smaller. This may require a specially compounded liquid form of the drug, to be measured in small, precise quantities.

Some other nutrients to use here are omega-3 fatty acids that help prevent brain zaps; magnesium 300–600 mg daily that has a calming effect; inositol 500 mg 2-3 times daily (in capsules or powder), and 2 hours away from the medication.

The rest is a similar program to the tranquilizer withdrawal covered in the previous chapter.

I will soon have a new Medical Food formula that helps with withdrawal symptoms as well, and shortens the weaning period.

SECTION 3

*Natural Ways
to Address Addiction*

Chapter 16
Breaking Your Addictions

If you cringe at the thought of stopping sugar, alcohol, and caffeine or if you're a smoker, turn to this section before attempting to wean off them. It will help you to understand the issues of addiction and its relationship to brain chemistry. You can then modify the detox to accommodate your imbalanced brain chemistry. You can still do the diet, but add in the suggested supplements to help with the cravings.

- Do you crave that first morning cup of coffee or really look forward to your coffee break?

- Do you find you can't wait to get home for your after-work drink and can't relax without it?

- Do you prefer dessert to dinner?

- Are you secretive about how much you smoke?

Whether it's sugar, caffeine, alcohol, soft drinks or tobacco, your dependence on them undermines your health. I seldom tell my patients that they "have to" stop or even reduce these addictive substances. The secret is that once you are on a well-balanced and nutritious diet and taking the right supplements, the cravings disappear! That's because they are symptoms of an imbalance that, once corrected, free you of the compulsion. You are then able to choose a drink with dinner or a cookie for dessert (and not a whole box of them, a sign of sugar addiction). Or not.

Now if you are genetically loaded for addiction, I would be more careful since many factors can tip the balance and it's best to abstain completely. However there should be minimal inner conflict involved here if you are chemically balanced.

Chapter 17
The Role of Toxic Chemicals
in Addiction

A big contributor to addiction is the toxicity in our environment, and as a result, in our bodies. Sad to say, we are living in a sea of poisons. We hear the stories on the news every day. Even the polar bears in the Arctic are loaded with mercury from eating mercury-laden fish. Inuit children have pesticides in their bloodstreams carried by air and sea and through the food they eat.

Newborn babies are shown to have high levels of chemicals in their systems. In 2004, researchers found a total of 287 industrial chemicals and pollutants in umbilical cord blood, including pesticides, consumer product ingredients and wastes from burning coal, gasoline and garbage in the blood of newborns. We know that 180 of these toxins cause cancer in humans or animals, 217 are toxic to the brain and nervous system and 208 cause birth defects or abnormal development in animal tests. These clearly pose a serious threat to the growth, development and overall health of these children.

The average American consumes about 14 pounds of chemicals a year in the form of food additives such as artificial food coloring, flavorings, emulsifiers, humectants, and preservatives. Then, beyond the known "bad stuff" that we ingest more or less voluntarily, we are also exposed to environmental toxins caused by everything from contaminated food to air pollution and secondhand cigarette smoke.

There are industrial wastes, hydrocarbons, chemical fertilizers, and pesticides in our air, water and food supplies. And don't forget the hormones and antibiotics that pollute most of our meat and dairy products. Even generally healthy foods like fish can be a source of toxic mercury and long-term exposure to heavy metals can cause brain and nervous system damage.

All of us are exposed to some or even many of these toxins. Most of us are not sick because of them, but it's a fine line between "OK" and "toxin overload." Toxins build up in our bodies, stored largely in fat cells, and we may not even notice their effects for years. Then the load becomes too great, we become imbalanced and the scales tip, causing a wide range of health problems, including headaches, fatigue, muscle weakness and more. Your brain can become unbalanced and in the search for relief, you can become addicted to foods, or other substances. It's more complex relationship than that but let's just say that these hidden toxins can wreak havoc.

If toxin imbalance is a major factor in your symptoms, you'll want to explore these issues more deeply as I do in *8 Weeks to Vibrant Health*.

Chapter 18

Detoxification Program

One factor that helps to reduce cravings is boosting the body's ability to detoxify and eliminate stored chemicals, including nicotine and marijuana, as well as organic compounds (like formaldehyde and other VOCs or volatile organic compounds) which are stored in the fat cells. There are things you can do to speed up this process: exercise, sweating, drinking plenty of water and supplementing with extra vitamin C and niacin. Put these all together, and you've got a winning formula for rapid detoxification.

Most gyms have access to a sauna or steam room. This is a great opportunity to enroll in a regular exercise program. Then here's what to do:

- Take 1g of vitamin C and 100 mg of niacin.

- Go for a run or do any cardiovascular exercise that raises your pulse rate and stimulates circulation.

- Once you start flushing as a consequence of the niacin, enter the sauna or steam room. Your heat tolerance will be lower than usual, but stay within your comfort level.

- Take in a quart of water with some electrolytes in it (my fave is Ola Loa Repair powder in handy packets) and keep drinking it at regular intervals.

- Do this for half an hour every day.

Take other antioxidants as well, such as alpha lipoic acid, 100 mg twice daily (Brain Recovery PM Formula contains 200 mg daily). See precautions on tyrosine and D,L-phenylalanine for high blood pressure, phenyketonurics, and those with bipolar disorder, manic phase. Note that the Brain Recovery AM & PM bottles contain different ingredients, and the program is made so you need to take both for the complete program.

Chapter 19

Food Allergies

In addition to these chemical poisons, many people have food allergies or, more properly, food sensitivities, some of which they're not even aware of, since they are "delayed," i.e., not occurring at the time you eat the food, but hours or even a day or two later. Known as IgG-mediated sensitivities, they can cause a host of symptoms including anxiety, depression, addiction and even bipolar illness and schizophrenia.

The most common sensitivities are to dairy (generally the casein protein in milk) and gluten, the sticky protein in wheat and some other grains. There are lab tests for the IgG antibodies (allergic or sensitivity response) to the food, or you can just do a food elimination diet as part of your detox. It works well for my patients.

I have more details on this in my *8 Weeks to Vibrant Health* book [http://8weekstovibranthealth.com] and program. You can start treating them with the Detox Diet, next.

Chapter 20
The Basic Detox Diet

For the next week, stop ingesting the following products.
Sorry, but if you are truly affected, partial elimination
doesn't work. The first three days are the hardest. The
rewards are worth it!

- Refined sugars

- Alcohol

- Caffeine

- Wheat and other gluten products (barley, rye, oats)

- Dairy products

- Corn and all corn products, especially high-fructose
  corn syrup

- Soy (allergenic and most often, genetically modified)

- Canned and processed foods

- Food additives, preservatives, and artificial flavorings

- Hydrogenated and partially hydrogenated vegetable
  oils, including margarine, shortening, and most com-
  mercial salad dressings and sauces

You can eat the following:

- Animal protein: Skinless organic poultry, eggs and
  wild game

- Wild-caught cold-water fish: Not more than two servings a week

- Organic sheep and goat's milk products, organic yogurt, and organic butter

- Rice, millet, quinoa

- Vegetables (all except corn which is too starchy, and regular corn is genetically modified), organic if possible

- All dried beans and legumes

- Fruit (organic, if possible), fresh or frozen

- Extra-virgin cold-pressed olive oil, sesame, or macadamia nut oil for cooking

- Flaxseed oil for dressings

- Bottled spring water, which contains minerals not present in filtered water

- Fruit juices (diluted 50% or more with water), vegetable juices, herbal teas, rice milk

This diet will bring you back to simplicity in your eating patterns. It is not intended as a weight-loss diet, but you are likely to lose some weight. What will happen is that you will begin to clear your system of toxins and food allergies.

You'll likely notice an improvement in your energy levels and other symptoms as the week goes on. You will also be introduced (or reintroduced) to the taste of real, fresh, whole food, just as nature made it. Whether they are steamed, raw, braised, you will find a new delight in these simple foods.

If you experience flu-like symptoms in the first few days, don't give up! Among your toxins may be yeasts and parasites. When they are deprived of the sugars that feed them, they begin to die, releasing their toxins into your system and causing temporary discomfort called "die-off." If this happens, drink more water, add 1,000 to 2,000 mg more vitamin C as a supplement, and read the chapter on dysbiosis in *8 Weeks to Vibrant Health*, where you'll find a more rigorous detox program to overcome intestinal yeast problems. On the other hand, there is a good chance that this detox alone will take care of your problem.

Ann-Louise Gittleman, in her book *The Fat Flush Plan*, suggests drinking eight glasses of unsweetened cranberry juice diluted with water over the course of the day. The easiest way to do this is to put 4 ounces of cranberry juice in a 32-ounce bottle and fill the bottle with water. You'll need two bottles of the juice cocktail a day.

To add even more power to the cleanse, take 100 mg of the herb milk thistle (also called silymarin) twice a day to help support your liver in the detoxification efforts.

An important point here is to be sure you are having regular bowel movements. Many toxins are released into the bowel, so if it's not moving, neither are these poisons. If you're constipated, take more fiber from fruits and vegetables and you can add a teaspoon of psyllium husks to your cranberry juice, once or twice daily: first thing in the morning, or in the evening, between dinner and bedtime.

Continue with a minimum of eight glasses of water (or cranberry cocktail). The bottom line here is once you remove the toxic energy robbers from your life, you will have far more vitality. You'll stop craving the "bad" foods: we crave the things we're allergic to, since they can make us high. Gluten produces gluteomorphins, and casein, casomorphins, which act like food-born morphine, an opiate that is a powerful euphoriant and highly addictive.

Be sure to keep a journal, especially the food-mood-supplement-activity record. You will be able to look back and track your "good" and "bad" foods.

Starting Back: Food Challenge Test

The next step will be gradually introducing certain foods back into your diet one at a time to tell what effect they are having on you.

You may be feeling much better after the elimination phase of your eating plan. You'll start experimenting by eating a portion of a suspect food. For example, if you think you have a problem with dairy products, drink a glass or two of milk and record your state at intervals over the next couple of days.

Only challenge with one food at a time and space your challenges by at least 24 hours, preferably more, so there is no confusion about which food you are tracking. This takes into account the delayed sensitivity that characterizes many food allergies. This will probably take several weeks, but you'll be developing a list of your hidden food allergies that will serve you well.

Reassessment: If you're still having symptoms, you'll need to dig deeper into the sources of your food sensitivities. Progressively eliminate some of the basic foods that were allowed during the elimination phase and see if you get results.

Maintenance. Now that you've discovered your triggers, you can lighten up a bit on the program. You can fine-tune your personal program because you know what works. If you challenged yourself on a food and passed the test, add moderate amounts back into your diet, but probably not more than three or four times per week. Called rotation, this spacing of potential allergens makes them less likely to become problematic in the future.

Again, your journal should be stuck to you: Record all your reactions. Don't waste a minute of this precious opportunity to learn about your food reactions.

Nutritionist Tom Malterre's Elimination Diet is a wonderful program for successful detox, with all the help you need to walk you through it in the form of a book, videos, and other aids. Have a look: http://tinyurl.com/nwcrzw6

Chapter 21

Relaxing Naturally

Drink, downers, and dope work by promoting some or all of the relaxing neurotransmitter GABA, the feel-good, neurotransmitters dopamine, and the endorphins. However, these substances also can cause an imbalance in neurotransmitter and blood-sugar levels that can get you into all kinds of trouble, from emotional and mental impairment to frank addiction. There are healthier, more natural choices that achieve the same goal, but without the negative effects.

While the ideal is to be free of stress and therefore have no need to use relaxants at all, the reality is that we do get stressed and would like to restore balance. To do this, we need to:

- Balance blood sugar.

- Promote release of GABA.

- Support the release of dopamine and endorphins.

- Supply the appropriate nutrients to produce them.

Stress depletes the body of vital nutrients. The more stressed we are, the more quickly we become deficient, and the more of these nutrients we need. For example, we need B vitamins for a smoothly running nervous system and for adrenal hormone production. There also certain minerals that have a relaxing effect on the body and emotions.

As we have seen, alcohol, cannabis, and tranquilizers affect one or more of these keys to relaxation. As with Marcy and Gene, they create significant rebound or withdrawal effects. The result is a never-ending cycle of stress – but natural relaxants can help you break it.

Relaxing Naturally with Herbs

Nature has provided us with a number of safe, effective, and non-addictive compounds that relax both body and mind. These herbs are readily available and inexpensive, and most have passed the test of time. In fact, most of our pharmaceuticals are actually plant-based compounds that have been modified and refined for more specific actions. However, unlike drugs that simply address symptoms, herbs work more subtly to promote the body's natural functions. Still, herbs can have powerful effects on the body, so if you are pregnant or nursing, always consult with a physician before taking any herb.

Valerian: A favorite for the treatment of anxiety is valerian (*Valeriana officinalis*), sometimes referred to as "Nature's Valium." As a natural relaxant, it is useful for several disorders, including restlessness, nervousness, insomnia, menstrual problems, and "nervous" stomach. Valerian acts on the brain's GABA receptors to produce a tranquilizing action that is similar to Valium-type drugs, but without the same side effects.

Be forewarned, though – it smells like old socks! So hold your nose, and here's how to take it. Using standardized extract (0.8 percent valeric acid), the dose is 50–100 mg, two to three times daily for relaxation. For bedtime sedation to promote sleep, take 150–300 mg about 45 minutes before bedtime.

Another word of caution: valerian can interact with alcohol and certain antihistamines, muscle relaxants, psychotropic drugs, and narcotics. Those taking any of these drugs should take valerian only under the supervision of a health-care practitioner.

For information on using valerian to help in discontinuing tranquilizers, see below.

The next two plants are traditional sedating herbs that you will often find in combination formulas. Like many subtle flavorings, they add their own special qualities to the mix.

Hops: (*Humulus lupulus*) has been used for centuries as a mild sedative and sleeping aid – to calm nerves and induce sleep, usually in combination with other herbal sedatives such as passionflower, valerian, and skullcap. Its sedative action works directly on the central nervous system. The dose is around 200 mg per day but varies from formula to formula.

Passionflower: The mild sedative effect of passionflower (*Passiflora incarnata*) has been well substantiated in numerous animal and human studies. The herb encourages a deep, restful, and uninterrupted sleep, with no side effects. Passionflower has been commonly used in the treatment of concentration problems in schoolchildren and as a sedative for the elderly. In very high doses, passionflower has been found to be mildly hallucinogenic, though I don't recommend trying that. Dosage varies with the formula but is generally 100–200 mg per day of the standardized product.

Relaxing Naturally with Amino Acids

GABA: We've now heard quite a bit about GABA, the main inhibitory or calming amino acid and neurotransmitter. GABA also acts as a significant mood modulator by regulating the neurotransmitters noradrenaline, dopamine, and serotonin. GABA helps to shift a tense, worried state to relaxation, and a blue mood to a happy one.

When your levels of GABA are low, you feel anxious, tense, depressed, and have trouble sleeping. When your levels increase, your breathing and heart rate slow and your muscles relax, making it a welcome addition to any chill-out program.

While you can enhance GABA activity with herbs, as we've seen, you can also take GABA directly in powder or pill form – 100–500 mg two to three times daily, generally mid-morning, mid-afternoon, and, if needed, at bedtime. Despite claims made to the contrary (those who think it only happens in an inflamed brain) a review article on GABA by two psychiatrists at the University of British Columbia found that GABA is able to move easily from the bloodstream into the brain. In technical terms, inability to cross the blood-brain barrier is often an obstacle to a product's effectiveness. So it is most likely that the GABA you ingest will actually get to its target, the brain.

Taurine: An amino acid that plays a major role in the brain as an "inhibitory" neurotransmitter, taurine is known for its calming influence. Similar in structure and function to GABA, taurine provides a similar anti-anxiety effect that helps to calm or stabilize an excited brain.

Taurine has many other uses as well, including treating migraine, insomnia, agitation, restlessness, irritability, alcoholism, obsessions, depression, and even hypomania/mania – the "high" phase of bipolar disorder or manic depression. People have also reported getting a pleasant high from taking one or two capsules.

By inhibiting the release of adrenaline, taurine also protects us from anxiety and other adverse effects of stress. It even helps control high blood pressure. You may have noticed it as an ingredient in some of the energizing, high-caffeine soft drinks, to soften any overstimulation.

Vegetarians can be at risk for taurine deficiency since taurine is found in animal and fish protein, especially organ meats. A non-essential amino acid, taurine can be manufactured in the liver and brain from the amino acids L-cysteine and L-methionine, plus the co-factor vitamin B6. When there are insufficiencies, though, you are best to supplement directly with taurine. The recommended dose is 100–500 mg twice daily, and higher as needed, between meals for best absorption. It can be found in Dr. Cass' CALM Formula.

Action Plan for Natural Relaxation
You must, of course, begin with a solid base, with the Healthy Brain Diet/Brain Recovery Diet and basic supplement plan.

B vitamins are required for the nervous system to run smoothly and for the production of adrenal or stress hormones. As well, certain minerals – calcium, magnesium, and potassium – have a relaxing effect on the body and emotions. Stress depletes these minerals, leading to further anxiety. So make sure that you are taking enough of the following, especially under stressful conditions: vitamins B1, B3, B6, B12, folate (best as methylfolate), calcium, magnesium, phosphorus, and omega-3 fatty acids, such as fish or flaxseed oil.

In other words, balance your body and provide it with the fuel it needs so that any new mood-enhancing additions will be able to do their jobs.

Getting and staying relaxed may involve making some changes in lifestyle, like adding in more exercise, mediation, and yoga. Changing your chemistry is just as vital, and here's how you can do it.

Balance Your Blood Sugar: An Even Keel
There are three golden rules for keeping your blood-sugar levels even:

1. Avoid, or at least considerably reduce, all sugar and stimulants.

2. Eat regularly and emphasize low-GI (glycemic index) foods versus high GI (like sugar, white flour) to keep your blood-sugar levels even.

3. Take supplements of the "energy nutrients," primarily B vitamins and vitamin C, which help to turn your food into energy more efficiently.

4. If you are very stressed, or suspect you have a blood-sugar problem, you will also benefit by adding a once or twice daily dose of 200 mcg of chromium, a mineral that helps insulin to keep your blood sugar levels stable.

Mobilize GABA: The Big Chill-Out

The following herbs and amino acids help to calm the stress response and act as natural relaxants. The ideal daily doses of all of them are less when combined than when the substance is taken alone. These are all suggested ranges, since responses will vary based on your unique chemistry. Test your dose carefully, and increase as needed. Then, add in one new item at a time, and observe your response.

Since herbs are extracts, the dose will vary based on the percent of the marker in the standardized extract.

For coming off tranquilizers, alcohol, and marijuana, and for overall calming:

Dose, 2–3 times daily:

- Valerian: 50 to 100 mg

- Theanine: 200 mg

- GABA: 100–200 mg

- D,L phenylalanine to raise mood during alcohol and marijuana withdrawal (in Dr. Cass' Focus Formula).

- Dr. Cass' CALM Natural Mind, containing calming herbs and amino acids: 2 caps 2–3 times daily.

- Dr. Cass' Nightly CALM, with added valerian – 2 caps 2–3 times daily for added sedation e.g. at bedtime.

- EPA/DHA 1000 mg

- Milk thistle (standardized to 70% silymarin complex): 200 mg.

- Keep your blood sugar balanced.

- Consider a master combination formula, containing all of the above, including blood sugar balancers, Dr. Cass' Brain Recovery AM&PM capsules.

So, to sum up, you should take the following to chill out:

- A multivitamin supplying optimal amounts of B vitamins, vitamin C, with 200 mcg of chromium (or take extra for a month or two). (See Dr. Cass' Better Balance Multi.)

- A "chill-out" formula providing valerian, hops, passionflower, GABA, and taurine, as needed (see Dr. Cass' CALM Natural Mind).

- For a good night's sleep, take 150–300 mg of valerian about 45 minutes before bedtime, plus 50–200 mg of 5-HTP, and either Nightly CALM, all of which help you to fall asleep and stay asleep, and if needed, SleepCycle® to restore natural circadian rhythms.

I recommend starting one new product at a time, observing your response, and then adding in a new one as needed.

If you're combining them, consider the combined effects and adjust the doses accordingly.

Helpful Hints for Chilling Naturally

Meditation, deep breathing, and similar activities are very useful for all addiction recovery programs. Regular aerobic exercise also helps, so this is a great time to sign up at your local gym, start jogging or do yoga.

Acupuncture is a great adjunct to any withdrawal and detoxification program. Dr. Michael Smith pioneered a very successful program at Lincoln Memorial Hospital in the South Bronx, using ear acupuncture to treat heroin addicts who were having unusual difficulty detoxing. When visiting, I was amazed to see patients in acute withdrawal, sitting quietly, even dozing, with acupuncture needles strategically placed in certain points in the ear.

Check out the website of an organization that I helped start, the Alliance for Addiction Solutions (http://transformingaddiction.com), where you can find holistic addiction treatment centers that incorporate these modalities.

Now What? Following Up
Everyone is different, and programs should be tailored, using the supplements that are precursors to the specific neurotransmitter, as seen above, in the "Nutrients for Brain Recovery" section below, as well as on my website. Once you have successfully withdrawn, you can continue solely on the Brain Recovery AM&PM Formula for as long as needed.

Since the initial addiction problem was often due to inability to produce neurotransmitters, many people will simply continue to take Brain Recovery indefinitely. *In fact, it's an excellent all-round brain and health-enhancing vitamin program, and I even take them myself for convenience when I'm traveling.*

Chapter 22

Getting a Good Night's Sleep

When you're addicted or withdrawing from an addictive substance, sleep can be a challenge. A good night's sleep is essential to brain and body function, and it's important to preserve or regain sleep at all costs.

Sleep is a complex and dynamic process with its own rhythms. We need to experience all the stages of sleep including REM or rapid eye movement sleep, generally suppressed by sleeping pills and tranquilizers. Research shows that increasing REM sleep time is an excellent mood enhancer. REM sleep is also like running a cleanup program on your computer: it cleans up and reorganizes the loose ends of the day, and is vital for memory storage, retention, mental organization, new learning, and emotional balance.

REM sleep increases as the night goes on, a good reason to get at least 7 to 8 hours of sleep. Another reason is weight gain: insufficient sleep stresses the body, raising cortisol, which causes insulin resistance, adding fat deposits around your middle – belly, hips, and thighs.

Just think of all the prescriptions written for neurotransmitter-enhancing antidepressants, or sleeping pills, when the underlying problem is actually sleep deprivation. In fact, many of these drugs suppress REM sleep and reduce the supply of available neurotransmitters, thereby aggravating low moods. These drugs basically knock us unconscious, then rob us of our precious restorative REM sleep. They are a lost cause – disturbing your sleep in the long run, then you have to deal with very difficult drug withdrawal, which I handle in my practice regularly.

Some other sleep tips: Be sure to eat at least 3 hours away from bed time, and follow the Healthy Brain Diet. Don't exercise or watch stimulating TV shows close to bedtime. Take a warm bath, turn the lights low, and in fact, sleep in a darkened room, with a mask if needed, to allow maximum melatonin production. Take your individual supplement program is a great start. Take no stimulants like D,L- phenylalanine or tyrosine past 4 PM.

Specifics for sleep are the same as the list for coming off downers: calming amino acids such as 5-HTP or tryptophan, glycine, taurine, GABA, glutamine, hops, passion flower, glutamine, found on page 78.

Sleep Specific Supplements

- Melatonin: 3 mg at bedtime especially in those over 50

- 5-HTP: 200 mg at bedtime,

- Glutamine powder: 4–8 grams (1–2 teaspoon) in warm water.

Warning: Some people have a paradoxical response and become stimulated on glutamine, as it converts to the stimulating neurotransmitter, glutamate, in their system.

- Nightly CALM

- Sleep Cycle

The Dr. Cass Brain Recovery AM&PM capsules have been very helpful for sleep as well as for balancing the brain. I have at times has people augment the 100 mg of 5-HTP in the PM bottle, though I have had great results with just the 100 mg contained in the PM alone, as in Charles' case below. The AM bottle contain the more stimulating ingredients, while the PM capsules, taken with dinner contains more calming ones like 5-HTP, theanine, and magnesium.

After having been on drugs of abuse, especially stimulants, being sober may not be enough to recover fully in terms of mind, mood, sleep, and energy. Charles was delighted to find quite a shift within days of starting my Brain Recovery AM&PM program as he wrote below. In fact, he was able to apply for a job for the first time in many months, and got it! He's still happily working there, too, some years later. I always see gainful employment as a major sign of a healthy recovery.

"After months of sobriety from various stimulants, I was still sleeping poorly and felt exhausted. However, within a week of taking Dr. Cass' Brain Recovery formula, I was amazed to find that I was able to fall asleep easily and deeply. I woke up rested, and my energy and focus lasted all day.

"I noticed that I was dreaming, too, which I hadn't for a long time. I felt as if my brain was restoring itself!"

– Charles R., age 45

Don't underestimate the power of sleep and don't skimp on it: Good, restorative sleep will cure many ills – including to help you lose weight! The reason? Lack of sleep generates more of the stress hormone, cortisol (see p. 91).

Chapter 23

The Brain Recovery Prescription

Now you know the relationship between brain chemistry and addiction, and have learned more about your own brain chemistry. Let's see what to add to your program to first help stop the process if addiction is an issue, and then, how to bring your brain chemistry to an even better balance.

1. Achieve Optimum Brain Nutrition

A good diet and the right supplements provide you with the necessary building blocks for brain cells and neurotransmitters, which are the mood, mind, and memory molecules. You will also be able to balance your blood sugar, which acts as brain and body fuel. This helps you to break your dependency on substances that interfere with normal brain chemistry and deplete your energy.

It is vitally important to eat well in order to restore and maintain your brain function and remain substance abuse free. Here you will find a summary of good eating habits – the Healthy Brain Diet. You don't have to be in recovery to eat this way: It's the way we were meant to eat. This diet supports your brain function, energy, immunity, weight balance, and overall good health.

2. Get "fine-tuned" with natural supplements

The reality of day-to-day life is that you will likely become stressed out or otherwise unbalanced. You will learn how to use natural substances to help bring yourself back into balance.

3. Think positively

Chemistry isn't the whole story when it comes to feeling great. It's also about how we think. Ironically, while fear and anxiety seem to come easily, we often have to work harder to achieve happiness. Fortunately, you can replace negative patterns with a more positive and uplifting frame of mind – and there are specific methods to achieve this.

4. Adopt a mind- & mood-healthy lifestyle.

There are many ways to improve how you feel, specific lifestyle changes in the form of physical, mental, emotional, and spiritual exercises.

The Healthy Brain Diet

It is essential to eat properly in order to restore and maintain your brain function and remain substance abuse free. Here's a summary of good eating habits, what I call the Healthy Brain Diet. You don't have to be addicted to eat this way: It's the way we were meant to eat. It supports your brain function, energy, immunity, weight balance, and overall good health.

- Eat whole foods and fresh foods, organic whenever possible; avoid processed foods.

- Eat three servings a day of top-quality protein foods– fish, poultry, lean meat (free range), egg, soy, or combinations of beans, lentils, and grain

- Choose complex carbohydrates such as whole grains, vegetables, and most fruits, and avoid sugar and refined foods.

- Eat fish three times a week, or take fish-oil supplements.

- Drink at least a quart of water, if not two, day, either pure or in diluted juices and herbal or fruit teas.

- Minimize your intake of tea, coffee, and soft drinks.

- Eat lots of antioxidant-rich fruits and vegetables–at least five servings a day.

- Take these supplements:
  - A high-potency multivitamin and mineral formula with antioxidants.
  - 1–3 g of vitamin C.
  - Essential fatty acids

In addition to a multivitamin, multimineral formula, I suggest the following, **twice daily**, based on the results of your personal brain questionnaire. I have added the product(s) that contains these nutrients:

- **Chromium** (200 mcg) and **Glutamine** (500 mg and also as needed for cravings), to regulate blood sugar and reduce brain fog and cravings for sugar, alcohol, or drugs: found in *Brain Recovery AM&PM Formula*

- **5-hydroxytryptophan** (5-HTP) 100–400 mg divided between AM and bedtime, both for depression and sleep problems, to boost serotonin levels: in *Brain Recovery PM*, 100 mg. Add more if needed.

- **Calming Amino Acids:** Theanine 200 mg, **Taurine** 500 -1000 mg, or glycine 200 mg to boost GABA when anxious or irritable: *CALM Natural Mind,* or *Brain Recovery PM capsules.*

- **Calming Herbs: Valerian** 100 mg (or 100–200 at bedtime), **Lemon Balm, Passion Flower:** *CALM Natural Mind; Nightly CALM* also has valerian.

- Tyrosine (500–1000 mg) and/or **Phenylalanine** (500–1000 mg) to boost dopamine for enhanced mood and concentration: *FOCUS,* 2 caps twice daily or *Brain Recovery AM (tyrosine).*

- **Specific Brain Cell Nutrients** such as **Phosphatidylserine** (100 mg) and acetyl choline precursors, such as **Phosphatidyl Choline** or **CDP-choline** 500 mg, **Acetyl-l-Carnitine** (500 mg), and **Ginkgo** (120 mg) to enhance acetylcholine, brain blood flow and brain cell health: *Brain Cell Support Plus.*

- **"Adaptogenic" Herbs: Rhodiola, Reishi Mushroom** and **Eleutheroccus Senticosis** to restore adrenal glands burned out by long-term stress: *Energy Boost.*

- **Omega 3 Fatty Acids,** in the form of fish oil 1000 mg twice daily to help restore the cell wall in which neurotransmitters are made: *Super EPA; Brain Recovery Formula.*

- **Extra B Vitamins** (50–100 mg) and **Magnesium** 200 mg to handle the depletion due to addiction and stress. They are essential in producing the neurotransmitters: *Brain Recovery AM&PM Program.*

Nutrients for Brain Recovery

To make it simple, I created a system of specific encapsulated formulas that work together to enhance brain function, which I included previously, but here they each are with full description:

1. Dr. Cass' Brain Recovery AM&PM Program™

The **AM Formula** ("Wakes You Up") is taken with breakfast and the **PM Formula**, ("Relax & Unwind") with dinner. Here is what they contain, with more details on www.cassmd.com:

1. High quality, high potency broad-spectrum multi-vitamin and mineral formula that provides the essential nutrients and co-factors needed to balance and restore body and brain chemistry.

2. Nutrients that diminish sugar cravings, encourage fat loss, and aid in preventing age-related changes, including Alzheimer's disease and dementia.

3. High dose of one of the most potent antioxidants and liver support nutrients, alpha lipoic acid, essential for neutralizing free radical damage to the cells and restoring liver function.

4. Precursors (5-HTP, tyrosine, glutamine,) and supportive nutrients (B6, Biotin, other vitamins and minerals) to optimize neurotransmitters.

5. Essential fatty acids (EPA, DHA) essential for formation of brain cells and neurotransmitters, and a key nutrient for healing depression, mood and attention

problems. They combat inflammation, improve cardiac function, enhance immunity, and balance hormones. This is found in Dr Cass' Super EPA, which is high potency and free of pollutants such as heavy metals.

Actions: Controls cravings and restores brain chemistry in substance abuse recovery. Also excellent for ADD/ADHD, anxiety, and depression, which have similar imbalances of neurotransmitters.

Recommended Usage: Start with the **Brain Recovery AM&PM** Program for 2 to 3 weeks so your body can adapt, and you can observe the results. After that, add in the specific 'extras' as needed. After 12 weeks on the full program, you can taper down the extras by 1/3 to 1/2 as a maintenance dose, while taking the packets indefinitely as your daily health booster. Many of my patients have found this program to be life changing.

2. Dr. Cass' Brain Cell Support Plus Formula™

- Powerful revitalizing nutrients for brain protection and brain blood flow

- Restores and maintains brain cell function for optimum mood, cognition and memory

Some of these nutrients can be felt within several hours (gotu kola, acetyl-l-carnitine), and others (phosphatidyl-serine, ginkgo) over months, as they gradually restore your brain cells. The ginkgo and vinpocetine enhance brain blood flow.

3. Dr. Cass' CALM Natural Mind Formula™

- Safe and effective replacement for drugs and alcohol: Calms your mind and relieves stress – without side effects, impairment, drowsiness, or loss of judgment

- Restores your brain chemistry (especially GABA) rather than depleting it.

- Enhances mood and sharpens mental acuity

4. Dr. Cass' Nightly CALM Natural Mind Formula™

Same as CALM but with added valerian, a proven non-addictive, hangover-free herbal sedative.

5. Dr. Cass' Energy Boost Formula™

- Combination of amino acids, minerals, and adaptogenic herbs

- Enhances feel-good, energizing neurotransmitters

- Contains adaptogenic herbs that support the adrenal glands – the core of your energy system – to boost energy, focus, and endurance.

6. Dr. Cass' FOCUS Formula™

- Acts like a cup of coffee, but without the letdown, addictiveness, and other downsides.

- Promotes mental clarity, alertness and a positive mood state without the side effects of herbal or prescription stimulants.

- Perfectly balanced blend of amino acids, vitamins, minerals and antioxidants that produces the two major mood- and attention-enhancing neurotransmitters, norepinephrine and dopamine.

Chapter 24

Recommended Program

For brain chemistry imbalance, begin with the **Brain Recovery AM&PM Program**

If you're experiencing sleep problems, add **Nightly CALM**. For problems with brain function, including memory loss and cloudy thinking, add **Brain Cell Support Plus.**

For added alertness and concentration, add **FOCUS**.

For adrenal support and sustained energy, take **ENERGY Boost.**

Most people find they do best when they take the whole system, since each component has its unique role. They all work well together, so there's no need to worry about negative interactions or taking too much.

Maintenance

You'll find that you can decrease your dose over time, but do stay on a maintenance program to keep your mind sharp, your moods stable, and to help prevent cravings that may lead to a relapse.

You can find more information about these formulas on my website, www.cassmd.com.

• For more details on the basics of brain function, see my book *Natural Highs.*

- You will learn about neurotransmitters, the brain's communication chemicals that are capable of stimulating and relaxing you, lifting your mood, and sharpening your mind.

- You will find out why some substances knock your chemistry out of balance, while others are good for you.

- You will discover the Natural High Basics, a core regimen of food and supplements that creates the best internal environment for sustaining mood and energy.

- You will learn how to support your brain and body chemistry for maximum energy and balance.

Since this program is a work-in-progress based on the latest research, don't be surprised if you see additional or modified products on my website where you can find more information about these formulas.

You have the information here to change your life forever. All you need to do is decide to do it. The rest will follow.

All the supplement formulas mentioned in this report are available for purchase exclusively on my online health store, www.cassmd.com.

Visit me on Facebook at www.facebook.com/hylacassmd and Twitter @hylacassmd

About Dr. Cass

Nationally acclaimed innovator and expert in the fields of integrative medicine, psychiatry, and addiction recovery, Dr. Hyla Cass appears often as a guest on national radio and television, including *The Dr. Oz Show*, *E! Entertainment*, and *The View*, and in national print media.

She has been quoted in many national magazines, blogs for the Huffington Post, and is the author of several best-selling books including: *Natural Highs*, *8 Weeks to Vibrant Health*, *Supplement Your Prescription: What Your Doctor Doesn't Know About Nutrition*, and *The Addicted Brain and How to Break Free*. She has created her own line of innovative nutritional supplements, available on her website, www.cassmd.com.

Diplomate of both the American Board of Psychiatry and Neurology and the American Board of Integrative Holistic Medicine, she combines natural medicine with modern science in her functional medicine practice. She has won awards for her contributions to the field of health care, from such organizations as Safe Harbor; the Orthomolecular Medical Society; and the respected Washington DC legal firm of Jonathan Emord and Associates.

A member of the Medical Advisory Board of the Health Sciences Institute and *Taste for Life Magazine*, she is also Associate Editor of *Total Health Magazine*, she has served on the boards of California Citizens for Health and the American College for Advancement in Medicine (ACAM). She graduated from the University of Toronto School of Medicine, interned at Los Angeles County-USC Medical Center, and completed a psychiatric residency at Cedars-Sinai Medical Center/UCLA. Toronto-born and educated, she now lives in Southern California.

Made in the USA
San Bernardino, CA
29 September 2015